Gone in a *Flash!*

10-day detox to tame menopause, slim down and get sexy!

Mari Carmen Pizarro, CHHC

This book is dedicated to women like me, who after a certain age didn't know there was a choice for vibrant health, a great body and a sexy attitude.

CONTENTS

PREFACE

Gone in a Flash! is a must-read for women who are ready to take charge of their health and reclaim control over their changing bodies. This book is for you if you are fed up with your current health situation, are in the preparatory stages of menopause, or are already menopausal. AND...you must be ready for change.

HOWEVER...if you picked up this book in the hope of finding a prescription for perfection or a restrictive solution guaranteed to solve all your physical and emotional problems—this book is not for you.

I am a recovering perfectionist and don't want to go there ever again. In my opinion, perfectionism is the religion of control freaks and insecure over-analyzers. Perfectionism led me to anxiety, paralysis, it stemmed from fear and was alienating me from the real world. Perfectionism is toxic—let's begin by letting it go.

This book will provide you with provocative information and will invite you to have fun exploring new ways of nurturing yourself. If you are ready to give your body a chance to reap the benefits of a clean diet, this book will inspire you to make simple non-perfect lifestyle changes, breathe a little deeper, and live freer.

ACKNOWLEDGEMENTS

My love, my husband, John M. Abt:

For allowing me to become whomever my heart desires—from corporate leader, to nutrition coach, to author. I know you unconditionally love and support all these crazy facets of my life. It is easy morphing alongside you; I adore you!

My children, Ana Sofia and Jose Francisco:

Because you continuously believe in me and never doubt the potential and desire to serve that burns deep within me. You inspire me every day.

My brother, Juan Pizarro:

For your altruistic dedication to my success. My website, my book cover, my image all represent who I am through your loving eyes and amazing talent. I love you, Bro!

My Lifestyle Coach, Nancy Reinhardt:

You kicked my butt when I needed it the most. Vision boards, time blocking, dedicated spaces, organizational techniques, a mission, and a crystal clear vision I will be forever grateful.

My editor, Heather Ruffalo:

Destiny paired us up; it was a hunch and I followed my heart. Thank you for giving me your best, guiding me, criticizing, correcting, and editing with love. Thanks for believing in me.

Joshua Rosenthal and Lindsey Smith:

For encouraging me to become an author. I still tingle with emotion when I hear your calling, your guidance, and your counsel. Your passion shines through, and it has definitely caused a ripple effect in my life. I am an author thanks to you!

My friend, Dr. Jonathan Wasserman:

For your creativity and commitment, for promptly and unselfishly replying to all my requests for help. For providing me the coolest book title, *Gone in a Flash!* and for the most thoughtful, sexy woman redefinition I have ever seen. You rock!

My muse, Natalia Rose:

You have been my inspiration and my guide. Ever since I read the *Raw Foods Detox Diet* in 2008 and later *Detox for Women* in 2009, I was transformed; you spoke directly to me, and I began to heal immediately. I promised to be your student, to learn from you, and to one day help others like you helped me. I am living my mission because you inspired me.

My clients:

Every day you confirm that I am on the right path. Each of you inspires me to continue growing, adapting, learning, and developing as a detox mentor and nutrition coach. Your honest feedback and loving praise keep me moving forward. This one is for you!

Introduction:
It Dawned on Me at 40.

Almost a decade ago, on the eve of my fortieth birthday, I was not happy with my appearance; I looked older than forty, I was more than ten pounds overweight and flabby, my skin color was dull, and my eyes looked tired. I thought a makeover for my birthday would be a great idea. I asked my husband at the time, Should I go for a fortieth birthday makeover and become a new woman?" He looked up, smiled ear to ear, and said, "That would be great, maybe shorter hair and new color!" I couldn't have agreed more! At forty I still didn't know that a new woman needed to come from within and had nothing to do with hair or makeup.

I happily went to see my stylist and shared my master plan to regain something I had lost. I wasn't even sure what it was, but I was sure I wanted it back. In the stylist chair, I happily shared my ex-husband's recommendation and demanded to be converted into a "new woman." She cut my hair, did lots of very blond, chunky highlights. I looked very different and felt great; I was a new woman!

Later that afternoon, when I proudly went to pick up my nine-year old daughter at school, I experienced an unexpected series of events. As I walked toward my precious Ana Sofia, I saw horror in her eyes. She started crying and ran back toward her teacher as if she had seen something really horrific. A very nice and empathetic mom looked at me said, "Hey, we have all done it. No worries; it can always be dyed back." Another, more cynical mom said, "Trying to be different? Won't work." Another said, "It's not that it's bad; it's just not you."

I was shocked!!! I wanted to say, "Hey, women! This was very expensive and well done!!!" But I kept walking toward my daughter while the teacher consoled her. The teacher was very nice; she assured Ana Sofia that all would be fine and this was just Mommy trying new things."

Two weeks later my hair was brown again. I was devastated. An expensive hair makeover didn't make me a "new woman." It had actually made me look older, and the lighter hair definitely didn't go with my complexion. I figured it was best to put this experience aside and move on.

I decided that since I was getting "old," it was OK to feel tired all the time, be bloated, look older, flabby, and not sexy. And how about those hot flashes? Oh well, they were hereditary, and I would handle them just like my mother before me did. After all I was forty! And how about my migraines, Irritable Bowel Syndrome (IBS), acid reflux, vertigo, and unexplained fainting? Oh well, this was my life. This was who I was. I needed to be strong and deal with it. There was no remedy for all this!

Other very unexpected and life-altering experiences were lurking around the corner. My very stable marriage and family life felt distant. My ailments were taking over me. I was dizzy, fainting, in pain, and in doctors' offices way too often. Life as I knew it was about to change.

I separated from my husband and moved from the beautiful

island of Puerto Rico to the US to pursue my executive career. But now I was a single mom who still felt sick, flabby, and older. I didn't have friends or family around, and I started feeling like I was fourteen again.

Wait...fourteen again!!!???

Yep. Very strange symptoms started to appear in addition to the stuff that was already bothering me. I was moody, hungry, gained weight easily, started sweating at night, my sex drive was not stable, migraines took center stage, my vertigo was constant, my menstrual periods were painful, and my hormones were messed up. I was not sleeping well. Pimples appeared along with an overall feeling of being spacey and ungrounded.

It felt like puberty all right but this time after forty. I remember hating puberty; aside from the hormonal mess, I felt ugly and as if I didn't belong. I was going through it all over again.

This was the complete opposite of how I had pictured my life after forty. I had this image of living a glamorous life. Even after my divorce I thought I'd be single, sexy and mature, dating beautiful men, going to fabulous events, being slender and strong, traveling. You know, shit you imagine but never comes true.

However, God, the Universe, and Mr. Destiny had other plans for me. I was approaching the "pause of meno."

Along with my unsexy, premenopausal symptoms, those faint memories of wanting to be a new woman started to surface again. Waking up with curly hair due to night sweats and then not being able to fall back asleep, provided plenty of opportunities to surf the net.

What if I had a choice?

The thought was too powerful to even seriously consider it. Having a choice would mean that being a tough woman who weathers the storm was not necessarily the right answer.

I honestly didn't believe in choice but rather in destiny. My menu of options was impoverished, and I was OK with it. Somehow I kept searching. I read all I could about prepping and enduring the "pause of meno:" migraines, diets, sweaty nights, hormones, etc. I researched for at least one year, and I read many books. It was then that I discovered a very novel term—detox. Whole or holistic detoxification to be exact. This means it encompasses all aspects of your life, not only what you eat, but your home, surroundings, career, relationships, spiritualism, your thoughts and your physical self.

What was detoxification? Isn't the body equipped to detoxify itself?

In my search I stumbled onto the woman who changed my life, Natalia Rose. No pills, no powders, no calorie counting, no judgment, no complexity, no fear. Natalia presented a simple almost unheard of way of living that promised a slender figure, a happier you, harmony with the universe, change from within, great food in great quantities, wine and dark chocolate. And a happier you! (I know I already said that.)

I tried part of the formula for a few months—just the food part;

the rest was too weird for me. Interestingly, the cleaner I ate, the better I felt. And even more interesting, many ailments began to subside, including, with some supplemental help, my dreaded nightly global warming episodes.

This got me thinking and pondering for a few months. I did nothing but fantasize about the concept of change from within. What if changing from within was that magic formula I had been in search of? What if what I ate, what I thought, what I believed, and what I desired mattered?

What if I had a choice?

■Chapter 1
Puberty after 40?
Defining the "Pause of Meno."

The "pause of meno" or menopause occurs when a woman is ready to begin her life as a mature, independent, sexy, and strong individual. It resembles a butterfly's journey— transforming from caterpillar to cocoon to total and absolute beauty. Remarkably, the caterpillar must die for the beauty to emerge.

I remember when the word menopause was not to be said aloud. It was synonymous with old, flabby, not sexy, moody, bitchy, and "downhill from there." However, the truth is that menopause and its predecessor peri-menopause are natural parts of a woman's life cycle, not diseases; just like menstruation and childbirth are not diseases.

Technically speaking, it is the "cessation of menses," or the "pause of meno," or the end of the dreaded menstrual cycles. No more womanly eggs to watch out for, no more prepping, no more shedding the uterine lining, no more Premenstrual Syndrome (PMS).

The years leading up to our last period are known as peri-menopause or "pre-pause," and the "pause of meno" or menopause is when our menstrual periods stop.

The phase leading to the "pause" can be characterized by periods that stop for awhile and then start again. A woman is considered to have been through the "pause of meno" once a full year has passed with no periods.

The average age for the "pause" is fifty-one, however, for some women this happens in their early forties or even late fifties.

According to Dr. John R. Lee in his book *What Your Doctor May Not Tell You About Menopause*, the symptoms associated with the "pause of meno":

> are peculiar to industrialized cultures and, as far as I can tell, they are virtually unknown in agrarian cultures. In native cultures menopause tends to be a cause for quite a celebration, a time when a woman has completed her childbearing years and is moving into a deeper level of self-discovery and spiritual awareness.

So how come we have been brainwashed to believe that menopause is an evil and obscure transition to old age?

In my personal experience, the symptoms associated with the "pause of meno" are caused by a combination of a dirty toxic diet, an unhealthy lifestyle, environmental pollutants, too much coffee and alcohol, cultural views and taboos, unnecessary prescriptions to mask the symptoms, lots of creative marketing, lack of self-love, and fear.

■Chapter 2:
Exploring the Upsetting Effects of Peri-menopause.

Feeling bloated? Fat? Headachy? Hot flashy? Not sexy and sluggish? You are probably experiencing peri-menopause, the transitional time before menopause. It is also referred to as "the menopausal transition." This is the time leading up to your last period. During this time your hormonal composition changes; levels of estrogen and progesterone vary from low to high even in a single day. These changes may be responsible for your hot flashes, headaches, weight gain, intestinal sluggishness, mood swings, and lack of sex appeal.

Is this the way your body tells you how angry she is? Perhaps she is upset at the changing circumstances. However if you listen carefully and clean things up, she might be able to do her job expeditiously and without the bumpy side effects.

Let's explore the most common symptoms one by one:

Bloat: In the *Mari Dictionary*, bloat is defined as gassy, tummy feeling like a balloon, burping and farting, sometimes constipated, and kind of disgusted at the whole thing. It is also defined as a feeling of fullness or tightness in the abdomen that can lead to discomfort or even pain. It is usually the result of water retention, increased intestinal gas, or a combination of both.

But why?

Bloating can be caused by many factors such as diet and stress. But generally speaking for women around the "pause," it might be related to a fluctuation in hormones, particularly estrogen. Rising estrogen levels tend to cause water retention, which leads to bloating and that full feeling in your gut.

Keep in mind that during this period estrogen raises and falls. When it falls, it can result in lower levels of bile, a substance responsible for keeping the intestines lubricated. If you don't have enough bile, dry hard stools accumulate in the small intestine causing their fair share of gas and bloating.

Other very important contributors are bad diet and stress. A diet containing carbonated drinks of any kind, lactose containing foods, preservatives, and food without fiber will definitely aggravate this symptom. So will stress, eating without chewing well, swallowing air and obesity.

Weight Accumulation:

Feeling Fat: Is it possible to gain weight with no rational explanation? My mom suffered terribly during her pre-pausal years and into the "pause of meno" with horrific, excess belly fat. I mean, she looked pregnant! How could this be? She always told me, "My dear, every year you must eat less and exercise more." And that's what she did even though it wasn't working for her. I was committed to following her advice but was terrified to grow older because I was already quasi-starving myself and working out often at only forty years old! I used to think, what the heck will my life be like at fifty?!

But why?

OK, it is true that the hormonal rollercoaster that occurs during the years leading to the "pause of meno" might make some women prone to weight gain, especially around the abdomen, hips and thighs. However, hormones are not entirely responsible for the changes in your silhouette. Maturing physically, a changing lifestyle (kids going to college, change in career, divorce, sickness or death of parents), stress, and genetic factors are also part of this equation.

Without regular strength training, your muscle mass will diminish with age. Loss of muscle mass decreases your metabolic rate (the rate at which we burn calories) making it much more challenging to maintain your youthful weight. So eating as you always have will most likely result in weight gain.

Of course, genetics and stress both play a big role. If your parents and relatives tend to carry weight around the waist, there is a chance you will too. Keep in mind that unmanaged stressful situations raise your cortisol which in turn triggers the storage of fat. Pair loss of muscle mass, genetics, stress, and imbalanced "dancing" hormones and you have the perfect recipe for weight accumulation.

Headaches:

From migraines to tension headaches, I used to experience them all. The worse being severe migraines that were debilitating. So debilitating that many times I was rushed to the hospital to look for the tumor that was hiding in my head, which of course was never found. I never associated my headaches with the food I was ingesting nor the significant hormonal changes and stress my body was experiencing. In addition, I started getting headaches before and during my period. They would appear the first day and go away in about forty-eight hours. Something was telling me these aches HAD to be hormone related, but what if it was something else?

But why?

As you may have heard, hormonal changes have been linked to headaches and to the disappearance of them. (You may have experienced this during a pregnancy.) Women prone to migraines or headaches might get worse as a result of the hormonal changes that occur in preparation for the "pause."

The truth is headaches can be stimulated by a variety of other factors like stress, allergies, lack of sleep, certain acidic foods like chocolate and aged cheese, a high salt diet, preservatives such as MSG, gluten, soy, and other external factors. These stimulants are more likely to trigger a headache when your hormones are "dancing" up and down. Controlling the headaches can be achieved if you identify their source and eliminate it from your diet.

Eliminating dairy, gluten, sugar and most preservatives and then adding green juices did the trick for me.

Hot flashes and night sweats

Global warming acceleration in your zone of the world: You mean you're not hot?

I have very wavy, thick hair that I manage to transform into a beautiful, silky mane after about 30 minutes with my amazing blow drier. Waking up with damp, curly hair was not in my daily plans. How much was I sweating at night to wake up with curly hair?

I often woke up soaked, totally wet and clammy, absolutely not approachable, and extremely uncomfortable. Only to be cold later as the sweat evaporated, leaving me confused and even pricklier.

But why?

Even though hot flashes and night sweats are common in about 70% of pre-pause and post-pause women, a correlation of this condition to hormonal changes has not been proven.

However, some health care professionals such as doctors, naturopaths, nutritionists, and dieticians attribute them to the decrease in estrogen. Remarkably, when estrogen falls during the "pause of meno," the hypothalamus can be affected which can lead to the brain detecting an overabundance of body heat. So to counteract, the brain releases chemicals to help lower body heat. This in turn causes your heart rate to elevate and blood vessels to constrict to allow for more blood flow. It is this increased blood flow that causes your temperature to rise, thus the feeling of global warming around you.

If you are in the 70% that experience this type of warming, I have good news for you. Generally, leading a healthy lifestyle can keep these flashes at bay. You will soon experience this when you follow the steps in this book.

Grumpiness:

Wearing your grumpy panties...literally. Out of the blue, bigger panties felt like a necessity. Maybe it was learned and passed down from earlier generations, but I knew that at a certain age I would wear them, too. After forty I gave myself permission to wear big, baggy, comfortable panties... all the time! The bigger and more comfortable the panties the grumpier I became; it was the perfect and predictable equation. One day, I accidentally pulled an old thong out of the grumpy panty drawer and tried it on. Guess what? Even this made me grumpy. Go figure! My mood swings and overall blah behavior were taking over.

But why?

Blah behavior, grumpiness, and mood swings are all associated with the preparatory stages of the "pause of meno" when imbalanced hormones are "dancing" to odd rhythms. Once in the "pause," the hormones stabilize themselves, and the symptoms seem to subside. Again, scientists have not been able to find a link between these symptoms and diminished estrogen levels. However, it is likely that the array of dancing and shifting hormones disrupt the harmony of your inner-self, thus contributing to an overall grumpy existence.

These changes can be stressful and hard to manage, often leaving you feeling anxious or depressed. But please be aware that, generally speaking, these are temporary nuisances and in no way meet the criteria for a clinical depression diagnosis or (in my opinion) warrant the use of anti-depressants.

Somehow, women experience more episodes of clinical depression than men, but again there is no evidence to link this to the "pause." Please note that if you have had previous depression occurrences, you may be vulnerable to experiencing relapses during this stage of the "pause."

Lifestyle changes, a fresh approach to the "pause of meno," a diet full of high vibrational foods (raw food that increases your energetic vibration or life force energy), a renewed sense of self-worth, and reduced stress will be your aides for keeping these at bay.

Sluggishness:

You feel tired...**of everything**! I was not a morning person nor was I a night owl. Actually, I was not even an afternoon person because of the 3 p.m. slump I suffered each day. So what was I? A sluggish zombie-like creature? A poor soul tired out of her mind of everything around her? So sad!

But why?

Sluggishness, feeling tired, or having low energy during the day can be a side effect of adrenal fatigue generally caused by a stressful life, carrying extra weight, aliments, unexpected life changes, depression, and the like. When you experience chronic stress, it can cause hormone imbalances. These imbalances may even contribute to a deficiency of progesterone, which is the main hormone responsible for balancing and opposing estrogen.

It is also important to mention a very significant hormone, cortisol. Cortisol is needed for nearly all processes in your body, from regulating glucose levels, helping the kidneys to function, building muscle/fat, regulating blood pressure, and more. When your lifestyle forces your adrenals to produce excessive cortisol, your hormone dance gets off beat. Your system can no longer respond to its own signals effectively, thus you feel awful. If you pair this with the natural hormone imbalances characteristic of the "pause of meno," the scenario looks grim and gray. However, as you will learn in this book, simple yet impactful lifestyle changes will play a crucial role in managing this aspect.

In summary, some uncomfortable yet common changes that occur in women after forty are attributed solely to the "pause" when that is not necessarily the source of the problem.

The symptoms discussed in this chapter are the most common ones and are based on my personal experience. I recognize, after much research, that fluctuating hormones could cause these, however, a definite link has somehow not yet been established. Think about this: How come men who do not have hormone fluctuations like we do also experience these same symptoms when they approach their fifties? I am talking about mood changes, depression, decline in sexual energy, changes in skin, hair, energy levels, insomnia and headaches. This is something I want to explore in my next book. Maybe they have their own "**man**-o-pause!"

■Chapter 3:
Detox to Tame the "Pause?"

Is it possible to ditch these hormonal side effects naturally? Why should you consider detox to tame the "pause of meno?"

Yes! It is absolutely possible to get rid of many of the common menopausal symptoms naturally. I am living proof that a systematic approach to detoxify your life is the best way and should be your first line of defense toward a better life.

I recommend a holistic approach to detoxification. I know the word holistic might be overused and many don't even care for it; I get it. Bear with me here. Holistic means all-inclusive, well-rounded, universal, whole, all encompassing. It is not a fluff word, and in this context it means more than just food.

I see our lives as a magnificent expedition comprised of many journeys. It is generally unpredictable and accompanied by events that are exciting, boring, scary, dangerous, exhilarating, sad, and happy depending on the stage you are in. From the detoxification point of view, I want to stress that you can make this a clean *or* toxic lifelong expedition. Which will it be for you?

A clean, holistic expedition will not only ease the side effects of the "pause," but it will make maturing a blissful experience depicted by the best health and vitality possible.

Detox for menopause is simply the process of freeing your body of toxins and harmful substances that accumulate in the organs and tissues. If the detoxification is holistic then it will be ridding your entire life of toxic things including your thoughts, home, relationships, and of course, your physique.

■Chapter 4:
What are toxins?

Defining sources of toxicity or trying to classify and list them all is a daunting task that I will not attempt here. However, generally speaking, toxins are classified as follows:

- Food toxins: Even in plant foods we find pesticides, herbicides, fungicides and genetically modified seeds. In animal products we find many of the above plus hormones, antibiotics, mercury, genetically modified species, disease and uric acid.

- People: We humans are capable of feeling, sensing, and experiencing a wide range of emotions. Some are very good for our soul and others very damaging and toxic such as envy, greed, discrimination, obsessiveness, paralyzing perfectionism, anger, fear, and judgment. The negative emotions are driven by deep-rooted insecurities that we often carry from the time we are born and contribute to a toxic existence.

- Environmental toxins (pollution): Pollution means that contaminants have been introduced into a natural environment causing adverse changes. Pollution can include chemical substances, sources of energy, noise, and gas. It is certainly difficult to move away from all environmental toxins, but a clean body with a strong immune system will be able to fight them commendably.

- Naturally occurring toxins: These are chemicals and substances produced by nature or by natural organisms that might not be harmful to the organisms themselves but can be toxic to humans. Examples are the fungus found in peanuts and some other nuts and naturally occurring toxins in shell fish and mushrooms, to name a few.

• Dietary Supplements: Nutritional supplementation is often necessary, especially during the preparation for the "pause" and certainly after the "pause" itself. However, some of these products have the potential to be counterproductive and actually contribute to your toxic internal environment. Did you know that the term "dietary supplement" was defined by *congress* in the Dietary Supplement Health and Education Act? A dietary supplement is supposed to be a product that contains ingredients aimed at supplementing an already good diet. (No supplement will detox you from a bad diet.) These products include vitamins, minerals, amino acids, probiotics, herbs and botanicals and are considered "foods" by the Food and Drug Administration (FDA) rather than drugs, thus being subject to lesser controls. Dietary supplements do not need FDA approval to be marketed nor do companies need to provide evidence that the product is safe or effective. My advice? Use with care and do responsible research before ingesting them. In my own research— and having used my body as a lab—I have found a correlation between the cost of the supplements and the quality you receive. Just saying.

Real life example: The National Cancer Institute decided to evaluate Aloe Vera due to its widespread use and concern that some components may cause cancer. After a two-year study of a non-decolorized whole leaf extract, proof was found of carcinogenic activity in male and female rodents. Scary! Carefully check all supplements before ingesting.

- Food ware: According to the Center for Food Safety and Applied Nutrition toxic elements and radionuclides are among contaminants of concern. They are present in some containers or utensils that come in contact with foods. Examples are glazed ceramic ware and silver-plated ware, many manufactured in China. Many plastic bottles and carton containers also have these contaminates.

- Household radiation: We are surrounded by radiation emitting products from medical devices to safety in airports and office buildings. Our homes are not exempt. At home we find the following radiation emitting convenient products: microwave ovens, cell phones, electric blankets, some anti-theft systems, remote controls, video monitors, ultrasonic toothbrushes among others. Awareness is key! Do without those that are not indispensable.

■Chapter 5: Are Chemical Toxins Really Part of the Problem? You be the Judge.

Did you know there are roughly 100,000 synthetic chemicals found in everyday items? Items like cleaning products, shampoo, booty wipes, carpet and upholstery, body creams, face creams, soap and bath gels?

The sad part is that many of them have never been tested for toxicity. And the ones that have may contain potential carcinogens and endocrine disruptors that are approved for use by the FDA.

 According to the National Institute for Environmental Health Sciences, endocrine disruptors are chemicals that may interfere with the body's endocrine system and produce adverse developmental, reproductive, neurological, and immune effects in both humans and wildlife. They exist in substances, both natural and manufactured, including pharmaceuticals, dioxin and dioxin-like compounds, polychlorinated biphenyls, DDT and other pesticides and plastics. And we find these disruptors in many everyday products including plastic bottles, metal food cans, detergents, flame-retardants, food, toys and cosmetics.

Did you know that on average one in three products we use for our skin and many anti-aging creams contain ingredients already identified as possible human carcinogens?

Become a smart consumer—be the judge!

This section is about awareness—not to be taken lightly but also not to scare you into thinking a bubble is needed to survive in this world. Humans are strong and our systems are highly adaptable. But the truth is we live in an environment saturated with chemicals that we are not designed to deal with.

It is not a surprise that after more than forty years of existence, our bodies, female or male, start protesting loud and clear for us to take action and remove what's preventing them from operating at their best.

If you want to learn more, check out the Centers for Disease Control (CDC) and Prevention's National Report on Human Exposure to Environmental Chemicals. The report is fascinating. Below is an excerpt for informational purposes.

> In the latest report, scientists at the CDC found that nearly every person they tested was packing a host of nasty chemicals, including flame retardants stored in fatty tissue and Bisphenol A, a hormone-like substance found in plastics, excreted in urine. Even babies are contaminated. The average newborn has 287 chemicals in her umbilical cord blood, 217 of which are neurotoxic (poisonous to nerves or nerve cells).

Did you know that we are exposed to more environmental toxins in one day than our grandparents were in an entire lifetime?

As I said before, I am just stating a few facts to get your awareness level up.

My goal?

Have you be the judge.

■Chapter 6:
Why do I Need to Detox?
Isn't my Body Able to Detoxify by Itself?

Do you remember when you got your very first car? Picture how exited you were to own your own vehicle. This one was one hundred percent yours. This vehicle would be your transport to go everywhere you needed to go. It would take you to school, to work, to beautiful vacation spots, to the hospital, to your wedding, to funerals, to parties; it would take you everywhere. All you had to do was care for it, clean it, change the oil and filters, replace the tires and put the right fuel in it, for as long as you owned the car.

I want to inspire you to think and feel about your body the way you did your first car. Except this time, the "vehicle" must last your entire lifetime, so care for it properly.

Questions I get a lot are: Why do I need to detox? Isn't my body able to detoxify by itself? And why complicate life now when dealing with the symptoms of the "pause" is more important?

Yes, your body is able to detoxify itself. Furthermore, your body is designed to get rid of and attack toxins and harmful bacteria. However, this precious vehicle and its Creator never predicted the need nor equipped us to get rid of the excessive amount of toxic waste we "ingest" on a daily basis.

You will see in the next chapters that toxins such as some of the food you eat, environmental pollutants, cancer-causing chemicals, preservatives, alcohol, man-made food, pesticides, heavy metals, and industrial waste have serious effects on your metabolism, behavior, mood, energy levels and immune system. Pair this self-induced toxicity with changes in hormonal balance during puberty, pregnancy, hysterectomies, peri-menopause, and the "pause of meno," and the picture is grim.

But where is all this waste stored? This waste is stored in tissues and cells throughout the body, including the brain, gut, and key organs—often for years. This is part of the reason we get worse as we age. It is not the aging itself but rather waste accumulation. Yuk!

Let us now shift our attention to some of our main detoxifying organs using the car analogy.

DIGESTIVE SYSTEM:

Where we add gas = mouth
Pipe that goes from filler to tank = esophagus
Gas tank = stomach
Oil = our precious blood
Exhaust system = intestines
Exhaust = rectum
A car's exhaust system works like our intestines removing yucky waste so that the car stays healthy.

Your digestive system (the esophagus, stomach, small and large intestines) is comprised of tubes through which orally ingested foods pass. These tubes are made of layers of soft tissue that absorb substances that are good or bad, depending on our eating habits. Did you know that the intestines are composed of four layers? If we separate each one of those layers, we will have approximately 250 meters of tissue—enough to cover a regular-sized American tennis court.

With a questionable diet, these internal pipes become clogged or corroded. Unless your food intake has been one hundred percent perfect your entire life, it is likely you have some junk built up inside you by this time. And believe me, with all the changes going on, you don't want clogged or corroded systems.

Then you have the LIVER which is the largest organ inside you, and the KIDNEYS which are workaholics. Both act as filters and are amazing creations of nature.

Did you know? Given the right internal environment, your liver could re-build itself, even if only 25% of it is still healthy?

Your liver goes into action every time you ingest something. Once your food and drink are digested, the good nutrients and the toxins (The liver doesn't discriminate.) enter the liver for processing. Depending on the level of nutrients in your meal, the liver will release the good ones to your blood stream or hold them for when you need a boost. If what you eat is toxic, full of hormones and antibiotics, high in alcohol, sugar or salt, the liver works overtime to try to remove or destroy the offenders. All these undesirable substances and toxins are then moved to your intestines or kidneys to be discarded. This causes the already busy organs to work overtime and tax your energy stores and digestive system.

Keep in mind that the liver also plays a crucial role in the body's use of hormones. Therefore, maintain a healthy liver by following the principles in this book. Limiting alcohol intake is central to maintaining a healthy hormonal balance, which in turn, is key as your body goes through all phases of the "pause of meno."

The kidneys, your two marvels that filter blood 24/7, can also produce hormones that alter your blood pressure. When your system is full of toxins and constricted, the kidneys get worried that there might not be enough pressure to take blood to all parts of your body. Intelligently, they produce a hormone that constricts the arteries (high blood pressure) to make sure that blood gets to all parts of the body. Most blood pressure medications work to block this function, thus affecting proper kidney functioning. All you need is the right diet (fuel) and exercise program (movement) to keep the kidneys working properly.

The Respiratory System's main function is to supply oxygen to all parts of your body. This system operates under the assumption that you inhale oxygen-rich air (which is not always the case), and then through exhalation, it pushes out air filled with carbon dioxide—a waste gas.

If the respiratory system is not working correctly or if there is an obstruction or toxic matter, the body will have trouble taking in air—like an asthmatic gasping for air.

The LUNGS are the air filters and the organ that benefits the most from exercise. Exercise makes the muscles around your lungs work harder and makes them stronger. Did you know that lungs are the "liver" of the respiratory system?

These organs, and others not covered here, were not created

to withstand a poor diet, sedentary life style, and toxic environment in which we now live. Yes, these are all built-in detoxification organs that are workaholics, self-regenerating, quality control agents, extremely loyal and dedicated to their jobs. But sometimes, perhaps by ignorance, we impair them from performing effectively.

■Chapter 7:
What about Hormone Replacement Therapy (HRT)? Can it be the Answer?

The HRT story is sad and disappointing, however, it speaks loudly about an era and a culture covering more than fifty years of medical history. It was an era in which aging was feared and a culture in which older women took the back seat in society. It was also the perfect time for sensationalism; marketing was on the rise, and the public was eager to try all things new—the microwave, canned meats, TV dinners, HRTs.

I feel it is important to explain where HRT began and to give you an overview of the many research mistakes, omissions, and the naïveté and narrow mindedness of some of the researchers.

Back in the 1920s, the use of non-contraceptive estrogen was promoted to handle the side effects of the "pause." And that might have had some merit in a few cases. But how can we explain why this one particular estrogen product became one of the most prescribed meds in the US during the 80s and 90s? Marketing geniuses, that's how.

It all began as a short-term solution to manage the side effects of the "pause" and transitioned to a long-term drug used for life after menopause to prevent, manage, and control heart disease, promote strong bones and avoid osteoporosis, promote a youthful appearance, and even to control mood swings. Or so they believed.

Slowly menopause became more and more medical and pathological as pharmaceutical companies, marketers, and doctors created a new market segment composed of women over fifty who were facing a life plagued by heart disease and osteoporosis. The only "cure"—HRTs. Let's not forget to add that to deal with the side effects of the synthetic hormones and excess estrogen that came along with HRTs, women were prescribed antidepressants. Have you ever educated yourself on the side effects of these drugs? Please do. You will be amazed.

Honestly, at the time, women were the perfect recipients for this miracle remedy combo. Researching a drug before ingesting, doubting your physician, getting a second opinion, trying alternative medicine, or going against the current was not in the cards. Women, including my mother, were "advised" by their doctors to take action with this miracle treatment. The alterative was a life with heart disease and osteoporosis. HRT was about hope. The industry cleverly associated synthetic hormone replacement with anti-aging, the fountain of youth, and the source of true beauty. I honestly feel I would have been prey to this scam.

Unfortunately, it was a few decades later that studies found evidence that this miracle drug could be to blame for increased risk of endometrium, breast and ovarian cancers, as well as heart disease in women using it for extended periods of time.

Two considerably large HRT studies were completed in the 1990s. One was a clinical randomized trial in the US (Women's Health Initiative) and one was an observational study in the UK (The Million Women Study).

The results of both studies raised serious concerns about the safety and efficacy of HRT.

These concerns pointed to two main issues:

- extended use of HRT may increase the risk of breast cancer
- use of HRT may increase the risk of heart disease

Enough said.

■ Chapter 8:
Can food be to blame?
Understanding food toxicity.

Food that is plagued with toxins and impurities accumulates in your body from the moment of your conception till the day you die. Toxic substances that moms eat when pregnant and while breastfeeding are the beginning of a potentially toxic life. Then you have the water supply, foods weighed down with chemical colors, flavors, preservatives and additives found in many baby products including natural baby formula.

Before we go into the steps to reduce your toxic existence through detoxifying methods, let us take a look at what "safe" and "natural" really mean.

How do we know if a product is safe? In keeping with the theme, I decided to research the Food and Drug Administration (FDA) database to find out what they recognize as safe.

The FDA has a Generally Recognized as Safe (GRAS) Notification Program. This is their definition:

> Any substance that is intentionally added to food is a food additive, that is subject to premarket review and approval by FDA, unless the substance is generally recognized, among qualified experts, as having been adequately shown to be safe under the conditions of its intended use, or unless the use of the substance

is otherwise excluded from the definition of a food additive.

The FDA is comfortable classifying a food item as safe (generally recognized as safe) by results of studies or through experience based on common use in food. In other words, if the food item or additive has been used with no side effects for some time it is OK, and if it has been studied it is OK.

According to the FDA, the meaning of "natural" on a food label is difficult to define. The agency claims that from a food science perspective defining a product as natural "…is difficult because the food has probably been processed and is no longer a product of the earth."

That is very interesting in a disturbing sort of way. How will we know if a product labeled as "natural" is safe? The FDA has not yet developed a definition for this term, however, they are OK with companies using the term as long as the food does not have added color, artificial colors, or things that are synthetic.

Big companies are very happy with this definition and use the "natural equals good for you" technique to manipulate people into buying their products. For instance, when an item is labeled "All Natural" it sends the message that it's good for you even if it contains lots of unhealthy sugars and fats. Very common examples of unhealthy "All Natural" foods can include most granola mixes, most crackers, most nutritional bars, most fruit snacks and most boxed cereals.

There are some fundamental questions not addressed in this generalization:

- Who is doing the studies?
- What constitutes a study?
- How often are these products studied?
- How long before requiring a study?
- Should we assume that no news is good news?
- What about studies that show sugar is addictive, inflammatory, and damaging for your overall health?

For those products that have been tested, the method used is called targeted chemical analysis. Targeted chemical analysis means to test for a *specific* chemical. The problem with this approach is that with more than 100,000 chemicals around, testing for all of them is nearly impossible. So how do we decide what to test for? For example, cyanide will not show in testing unless you are specifically looking for it. The same is true for most chemicals that circulate around our food with total freedom.

■Chapter 9:
The Skinny on Genetic Engineering a.k.a. Genetically Modified Organisms (GMOs).

A genetically engineered organism is born when scientists introduce new qualities or characteristics to the DNA of an organism like a plant cell. A common example is seeds. Seeds may be genetically engineered to produce qualities that enhance growth, change the nutritional value, or make them insect resistant. GMOs were introduced into our food supply in the 1990s.

The FDA has set up a voluntary consultation process to engage with the developers of genetically engineered plants or seeds to help ensure the safety of these products. Note—it is *voluntary,* not required.

From a government's perspective, how is the safety of food from genetically engineered seeds evaluated? According to the FDA, the developer identifies the new genetic characteristics and assesses if the new material could be toxic or allergenic. How the developer does this is up to the individual developer. Then a team of scientists from the FDA evaluates the report submitted by the developer. The consultation is deemed complete when these scientists are pleased with the developer's safety assessment.

Unfortunately, I have not been able to find an individual source of data (at least not funded by the developer) explaining how these evaluations are made. And I have a few questions yet to be answered:

- What happens when a plant cell is genetically engineered to contain insecticide/pesticide/herbicide properties in its DNA?

- How does the group of scientists in the FDA validate that this is not a safety concern in the long run?
- What studies are being undertaken to ensure that no long-term effects are to be experienced from exposure to insecticide or toxin producing crops?

One of the most widely used GMO seed is the weed killer resistant variety. This means the plant cell has been engineered to be resistant to powerful weed killers allowing farmers to use massive amounts of chemicals to effectively kill weeds. When farmers spray massive amounts of weed killer on their crops, there is a big chance that it will end up in our fruits and vegetables.

An interesting detail is that between 1996 and 2008, US farmers sprayed an extra 383 million pounds of herbicides to their GMO crops. This massive amount of herbicide results in "super weeds" because only the strongest survive. Then more herbicide is needed every year, but the stronger weeds will survive and reproduce. Not only does this creates massive environmental disturbances, it puts higher levels of toxic residues on GMO foods.

Did you know that herbicides in weed killers have been linked to sterility, hormone disruption and birth defects? Again ladies, we don't need extra hormone disruption, so let's ban GMOs from our life. It is simple and totally doable.

For more information, refer to the American Academy of Environmental Medicine (AAEM). They have done a great job of educating doctors to prescribe non-GMO diets to all patients and conduct studies in an effort to obtain real, unbiased data on the effects of GMO foods in our diet.

■Chapter 10:
The Two Most Injurious Side Effects of Toxicity—Inflammation and Acidity.

If you are reading this, you are probably over forty. You have a hectic lifestyle, follow the standard American diet, don't move enough, are stressed, and are going through the prep for menopause. You are definitely in need of some serious detoxification.

Did you know that if you are eating a typical American diet chances are only 20% of your body's waste and toxins have been naturally evacuated and removed?

Imagine cleaning every room in your house but leaving trash in the hallways over a period of more than forty years. Yuk!

Have you put on weight so your body can accommodate the extra waste? How is your energy level? Can you trust that your body will take you to all the places you want to go until you leave this world? Your cell function is impaired when they are clogged and cannot release waste.

Using this program to detoxify your cells will improve your ability to absorb nutrients and eliminate waste. This is the first step to tame the symptoms of the "pause."

Did you know that when your body is incapable of eliminating waste it becomes acidic? An acidic body is toxic. When our vessel is toxic, all rebuilding processes within slow down. When this happens, your body starts to slowly break down.

Toxins accumulate when you ingest more food items than you can eliminate. This goes for food and external toxins, as well as, feelings of stress and being overwhelmed. When this happens, you inhibit your body from being able to deal with the necessary preparations and changes for menopause.

When we don't do a detox regularly, the acidity of our diet promotes the growth of micro-organisms (yeasts, molds, fungi) and produces Mycotoxins, which in turn create more toxins. These toxins are stored in our cells. Keep in mind that the quality of your life depends on the quality of your cells.

How can we keep our cells healthy? Cells have very basic needs for their survival—oxygen, water, clean fuel, and a functioning elimination system. This 10-day detox plan is intended to help you improve the quality of your cells by focusing on these same areas—receiving oxygen and clean fuel, being properly hydrated, and ensuring proper elimination.

Inflammation

Inflammation is one of the underlying causes of disease. It means holding on to excess weight, pain, heaviness in the abdomen area, and excess heat in the body. Inflammation is basically a biological response that occurs to protect the body from pathogens, damaged/clogged cells, or external irritants. Inflammation is a defense mechanism tasked with removing the offensive intruder and beginning the healing process. This is one of your body's methods of communication. Are you paying attention?

Don't run yet; there is good news. You can manage this, but you need to commit to listening to your body and deciding to take an active role in its detoxification process. I promise you nobody will do this for you. This one is on you!

What other offenders contribute to inflammation? Some other causes of inflammation are sugar, lack of exercise, food allergies, food sensitivities, excessive stress, and alcohol.

Did you know that inflammation alone causes weight gain and prevents weight loss? So when we are inflamed, we get fat and being fat provokes inflammation.

Acidity

This might come as a shocker to you, but if we could rewind the tape of our existence a few thousand years, we could confirm that all humans were created equal. Yep, all with the same operating system, the same biological needs, the same parts, the same chemical lab...you get the point.

We are designed to thrive in alkaline environments, both internally as well as externally, versus the acidic epidemic in which we exist today.

Let me explain what I mean by an alkaline environment:

You might recall when your middle school chemistry teacher

attempted to teach you about acids and alkalis using pH strips. It goes like this: pH is measured to determine how acidic or alkaline a substance is and provides us with a numeric range from 0 to 14. Acidic substances range from 0 to 7 and alkaline substances between 7 and 14.

If we measure human pH in a clean, biological, non-toxic state, our body falls in the pH range between 7.35 and 7.45 which makes us naturally alkaline. When we eat, think, breath, or live in acidic environments, we are tipping our pH out of its natural range and setting the stage for poor health and hormonal imbalances. Foods like non-organic meat and dairy and eggs, soy products, gluten, man-made concoctions and alcohol, contribute to an internal acidic environment. When we become acidic, our system will work to bring us back to balance, back to homeostasis. It will work hard, and it will make this task a priority leaving no time for anything else. No time to battle infections efficiently, no time to naturally detoxify properly, no time for adequate digestion, no time to rebuild and prepare us for the "pause of meno."

Overall body toxicity in the form of inflammation and acidity will eventually disrupt your thyroid function, ruin female hormone balance, and may account for depression, anxiety, and fatigue. Is this making sense? Could it be that all we need to do is allow our system to get ready for the "pause of meno" in a clean environment?

Following the principles in this book you will be able to bring your system back to a balanced pH. As a rule of thumb, to be able to detoxify and balance your system, you should strive for a diet consisting of 80% alkaline foods and 20% acid-forming foods. These foods will be explained in the next chapter.

■Chapter 11:
A Jumpstart Solution.

You are about to learn the most important and easy-to-implement tool to jumpstart your detoxification process and conquer the "pause's" most annoying side effects. When you follow these principles you will see changes in as little as 10 days, however, I invite you to repeat the plan two or three times to obtain beautiful, long-lasting results.

I love science, and there is science behind this madness. The scientific term is "trophology," which is the practice of proper food combining.

But before I dig in into which foods you should eat together and why, I want to introduce the following points:

- Learning how digestion affects our overall health, mood, energy levels, and mental agility is key to understanding why food combining is so effective.

- Transitioning to a clean diet is imperative for optimal results and must be the ultimate goal of any weight-loss and health-improvement solution.

- This chapter is intended to educate you in making easy changes to the way you combine your meals.

Food Combining: Overview and the science of why this works

Food combining is the first concept I introduce to all my clients and the key to all my detoxification processes. Even before I introduce clean eating, I want you to try combining foods differently. There is a lot of evidence to support food combining, and I feel blessed to have found this solution, as it has worked wonderfully at keeping the most common "pause of meno" effects at bay. Proper food combination has allowed me to maintain a healthy weight, superb levels of sexy energy, and a zest for life well into my 40s, and I enjoy a great variety and abundance of food. Good-bye tiny portions, counting calories, and hours at the gym.

The science behind it:

Trophology, or food combining, endorses specific combinations of food and nutrients in one meal as the key to good health. The main principle of proper food combination is not mixing carbohydrate-rich foods with animal proteins in the same meal.

Why? Well, acidic foods such as proteins require a different environment to be properly digested than alkaline (base) foods such as carbohydrates. When we avoid mixing them in the same meal, we enhance digestion, shorten the transit time for them to exit the body, and save tons of energy due to shorter digestion times.

Guess where the saved energy goes? You got it!

Basically, when food passes through our system quickly,

especially clean food, it literally cleanses your digestive track of old waste collected in the intestines. The result is less accumulation, no bloating, gas, or sluggishness along with a flatter abdomen.

The principles of food combining are not based on giving up certain foods but rather on eating them in a different way—a way that allows them to pass through and exit our system quickly.

The main challenge is that many of the foods we are accustomed to eating together during a normal dinner start shutting down digestion as soon as they are put in our mouth. This is why you might feel bloated, tired, and sick to your stomach after a meal.

It is the norm to combine "pasta with chicken," "meat and potatoes," "burgers and fries" or "eggs and toast." But what happens is that proteins and carbohydrates need different digestive enzymes to be properly broken down and absorbed. When we mix them, it takes our stomach longer to digest which allows food to ferment in our gut. When food ferments, digestion is stalled, and when digestion stalls, we hinder nutrient absorption and slow down the metabolic rate, thus interfering with our goals.

I will teach you a very simple way to still have most of the foods you love but organized in a different way. You will learn what foods combine well together so that your meals move quickly out of your body, retain the majority of the nutrients, increase your metabolic rate, and tame the "pause."

To make food combining easy, I have divided the foods we eat into 5 major categories.

1. Proteins: foods that contain 15% or more protein matter

   a. Concentrated proteins: meat, fish, fowl, eggs, milk, cheese
   b. Lighter proteins: nuts, beans, peas, soybean products

2. Starches (carbohydrates): foods that contain 20% or more starch and/or sugars

   a. Starches: peanuts, bananas, potatoes (all types), squashes, all pasta products, oatmeal, most grains, rice, breads of any kind, cakes, cereals, granolas
   b. Sugars: whole, brown and raw cane sugar, coconut sugar, fructose, honey, maple syrup, dried sweet fruits (raisins, figs, prunes), dates

3. Fruits:

   a. Acid fruits: orange, grapefruit, lime, lemon, all berries, cranberry, pineapple, tomato, passion fruit
   b. Sub-acid fruits: apple, pear, peach, cherry, grape, apricot, nectarine, plum, papaya, mango, etc.
   c. Melons: watermelon, musk-melon, honey dew melon, cantaloupe, papaya
   d. Exceptions: bananas act as a starch; avocados act as a fatty starch; dried figs, raisins, prunes and dates act as sugars

4. Fats: animal or vegetable oils

    a. Animal: butter, cream, lard, tallow, ghee
    b. Vegetable: olive, soybean, sunflower seed, sesame, safflower, corn, palm, and all nut oils

5. Neutral Vegetables:

    a. All leafy greens, celery, cabbage, broccoli, spinach, all spouts, cucumber, asparagus, onion, garlic, scallion, leek, eggplant, turnip, watercress, zucchini, string bean, pepper, radish, carrot, okra, artichoke, olives, beet, jicama, fennel, mushrooms, sea vegetables
    b. Exceptions: potatoes and squashes act as a starch

In the simplest terms, the most important principles to follow are:

- **Never mix starches/carbohydrates and proteins in the same meal.** Examples of good combinations are an avocado sandwich, veggie wraps, meat with veggies, fish with veggies or quinoa salad.

- **Don't be afraid of using good fats.** Use them to cook (ghee, organic butter, coconut oil), in dressings (olive oil, coconut, or avocado) or in smoothies (coconut or avocado) if needed for calorie maintenance. Remember you must include them to lose weight in a healthy manner, so don't be scared of them!

- **Neutral veggies can accompany any meal.** They are neutral and combine well with all categories.

Good examples are fish with veggies, quinoa salad, vegetarian lasagna or veggie stew.

- **Eat fruit alone or with neutral veggies.** For example use fruit in smoothies with neutral veggies or eat alone as a snack between meals.

I promise this is really easier than you might think. Overall, we want to aim for an alkaline/base environment within our body.

Don't panic, food combining really is easier than you think. I like to think about these categories as sports teams. Teams work very well together but rarely mix with other sports. Football teams don't play baseball teams, right? And in sports, there is usually a referee—a neutral agent—to ensure things run smoothly.

TEAM $\mathbb{N}$ = Neutral Vegetables (Referee)

TEAM S = Starches/Carbs

TEAM P = Proteins

TEAM F = Fruit

FATS/OILS = Use sparingly, combine as neutral

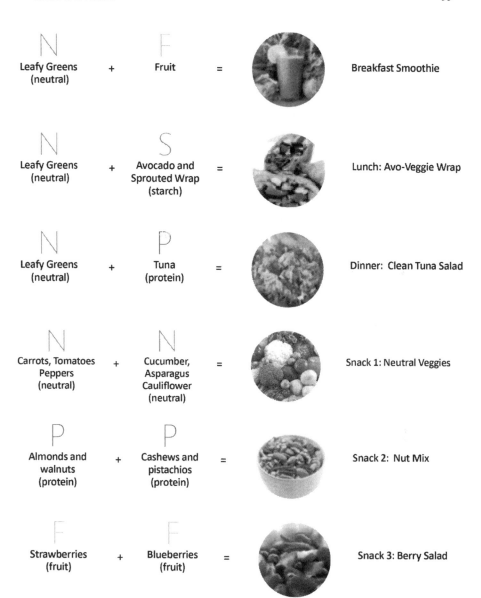

N Leafy Greens (neutral)	+	F Fruit	=	Breakfast Smoothie
N Leafy Greens (neutral)	+	S Avocado and Sprouted Wrap (starch)	=	Lunch: Avo-Veggie Wrap
N Leafy Greens (neutral)	+	P Tuna (protein)	=	Dinner: Clean Tuna Salad
N Carrots, Tomatoes Peppers (neutral)	+	N Cucumber, Asparagus Cauliflower (neutral)	=	Snack 1: Neutral Veggies
P Almonds and walnuts (protein)	+	P Cashews and pistachios (protein)	=	Snack 2: Nut Mix
F Strawberries (fruit)	+	F Blueberries (fruit)	=	Snack 3: Berry Salad

In summary, starches/carbs don't combine with proteins in the same meal, and neutral veggies go with everything. Eat fruit alone and fats only as needed.

Understanding food combination principles is the first step toward total body detoxification.

This is your detox jumpstart!

■Chapter 12:
Welcome to your Solution!
Your Symptoms Gone in a *Flash!*

This part is very dear to my heart. It was created in an effort to put all the detox components I have learned from many experts and my own experiences all in one place. You have done a lot of reading and now it is time to start making sense of it all.

Taming the symptoms of menopause holistically is the groundwork to overall well-being and radiance. You will experience a decrease in symptoms, increased energy, a better mood, and a slimmer you...naturally.

I guarantee you will use the information here as reference again and again until you attain a state of optimal wellness. As I approach the mid-life mark, I make a conscious effort to continuously follow the principles described here. And I feel better and more radiant every day.

Ready yet?

- Make sure you completely understand the principles of food combination.
- Set your goals and put them on your calendar. When are you going food shopping, what do you need buy, need any new kitchen equipment such as blender, peelers, mini food processor, box grater?

- Indulge in a few self-care items: candles, essential oils, incense, bath salts. This does not have to be expensive; a good quality relaxing oil and Epson salts create a luxurious bath experience for less than $0.50 per bath.
- Once you have what you need, get organized. Pre-wash veggies, organize pantry, make sure you have all you need to guarantee success.
- De-clutter your space and make sure you also remove temptations.

Note: I want to stress that the food part of this detox on its own is not the solution to all your problems. You must eliminate toxins and minimize exposure to new ones in conjunction with rebuilding the body with vitamins and minerals, as well as proper waste elimination.

This plan is gentle, short, and based mainly on eating whole foods that will jumpstart your journey to radiance. Whole foods are foods in their natural state—no processing, packaging, and minimum handling. Examples include fresh vegetables, bulk grains, fresh wild caught fish and nut butters.

It might seem difficult the first few days compared to the standard American diet, but I promise you this will pass. You will NOT be hungry, and you will start feeling good in two or three days. You will not be restricting calories, counting grams of anything, adding points, or working long hours in the kitchen. This is simple.

You might be wondering when the best time to detox is. *Now* is the best time to detox! I encourage you to commit to this program now. You will be eating whole foods, no gimmicky anything, therefore, you can do this while at work, while on vacation, if you are very busy, or if you are at a relaxed stage in your life.

I invite you to make whatever excuse you have to procrastinate the reason why to do this now.

Did you know that you can transform any procrastination excuse into the reason to take action? My client Sara told me she could not focus on herself now because she was preparing two kids for college and was too stressed. She was visiting schools, writing essays, filling out paperwork. She was exhausted, premenopausal, and frazzled all the time. How about this reframe: Because she must help get these kids through college, she must focus on herself, must increase her energy, and must be an example for them.

Please keep in mind that when you decide to embrace a healthier you, following this detox will slightly alter your daily routine because you will be doing things differently. But in no way will it interfere with your life. It will enhance it!

One thing you will notice is the amazing awareness that comes when you pay attention to what you eat. How different foods make you feel, how your taste buds will clean up, how your energy levels will go up, and how you will feel renewed both physically and emotionally. This awareness will also provide you a sense of control over your state of mind.

Determining your unique solution:

I will do my best to guide you through this process, but I want you to own it. Wonderful outcomes happen when you are empowered to take responsibility, listen to your body, and adjust as needed to fit your unique nature.

You will be doing this for 10 days, and I have divided into three stages: Prep Stage, Go Stage, and Consciousness Stage. However, you can lengthen it to a maximum of 28 days, which is the most effective way to go deeper and find that sexy mama that is hiding behind the toxic curtain.

I want to meet you where you are and allow you to adjust the number of days you spend in each phase. The guidelines below will serve as an aid to determine the length of your program.

10-Day Solution: This is for those of you who are already on a healthy path, you cook most of your food, avoid most packaged foods, evacuate more than once per day, read labels, eat out less than 3 times/week, are not addicted to coffee, have one or two drinks per week max, and would love to release less than 8 pounds.

21-Day Solution: This is for those of you who are seriously considering making a change to get on a healthy path but are not there yet. You cook occasionally, use some packaged foods for convenience, evacuate one time/day or less, read some labels, eat out more than 5 times/week, like your coffee but are not addicted to it, have one or two drinks per week, and would love to release 8-10 pounds.

28-Day and Beyond Solution: This is for those of you who know you need to improve your health situation but "now is never the right time." You rarely cook, are hooked on coffee, packaged foods are your staple, are constipated, rarely read labels, eat out almost every day, and would love to release 10-12 pounds.

Note: The program length that I use with most of my clients over forty is the 21-Day Solution detox. I guide them through the whole process and allow them to get into the best possible state. This longer program gets them ready to introduce juicing and colonics into their life, which is taught in my *Six Weeks to a Radiant You* program. The combination of these two programs produces astonishing results and improves all areas of their lives. For more information on this program please visit my website at http://www.streamlinedhealth.com.

By now you should have determined the amount of time you will dedicate to your detox. In the following chapters I will hold your hand to ensure a smooth transition and much deserved success.

■Chapter 13:
Shaping-up your Diet — Zapping and Adding.

Consider the following recommendations as the minimum operating requirements to get you closer to your goals: You already made a commitment, you are halfway through this book, you are ready. Let's get this done!

What you want to zap from your diet ASAP!

- You must eliminate milk from your diet. It doesn't combine well with anything and halts the digestion process. It isn't meant for human consumption. It's loaded with hormones and antibiotics, it forms mucus, and it's highly acidic for your system. If you must have cheese, choose organic raw cheeses (goat or sheep cheese) which are delicious and easier to digest.

- Ditch the soda/pop. Carbonated sweet drinks of any kind are horrible for you because they provide no nutritional value. And the diet versions are even worse; they trick your digestive system and make you crave more sugary drinks later.

- Stay away from processed foods including tofu. If a label has more than five ingredients and they are not recognizable as food when you read them, then your body won't recognize them either. Foods in this category are poison and are stored as toxins.

- Stay away from supermarket prepared foods or any diet pre-prepared foods. These foods tend to be loaded with preservatives, unhealthy fats, and even chemicals. Your system will have a hard time breaking them down which will cause fermentation and putrefaction. Opt for the salad/fresh bar instead.

- Try to avoid desserts right after your meal. Once you reach your ideal weight you can have sweets but try for natural alternatives like homemade ice creams, teas with raw honey, or dried fruit. But eat them an hour or two after your meal.

- Avoid alcohol, especially during your regular workweek. If you want to drink, have a glass of red wine and nurse it, enjoy it, savor it. Slow down! Wine combines well with most meals. (My advice is to go for the good stuff!)

What you want to add to your diet:

- Drink purified or spring water—lots!!! Water will assist you to flush impurities, keep you hydrated, and help you look younger. If you are not used to drinking plain water, a slice of lemon makes all the difference and will aid in the flushing of toxins.
- Buy organic produce. If purchasing all your produce as organic is difficult, aim for going organic for the "dirtiest" of all. *The Environmental Working Group*

(EWG) 2013 Shoppers Guide has identified the following offenders as the "Dirty Dozen™ Plus":

- o apples, celery, tomatoes, cucumbers, grapes, hot peppers, nectarines (imported), potatoes, spinach, all berries, bell peppers, kale, collard greens, and summer squashes

- Add high fiber veggies EVERY day. If your digestive system is healthy and unadulterated by surgery, fibrous veggies will help with the cleansing. They act as a broom, sweeping away waste. Examples of fibrous vegetables are broccoli, cauliflower, asparagus, Brussels sprouts, spinach, carrots.

- Opt for raw foods when possible. Load up on raw and fresh fruits and veggies when possible instead of the canned or packaged options.

- Eat double duty foods. Quinoa, for example, (more a seed than a grain) offers a healthy amount of complex carbohydrates along with a decent amount of protein and fiber. The same is true for chia seeds.

■Chapter 14:
Detox Stages—What to Expect.

In all stages you will experience mild to bothersome adjustment symptoms. You are changing the way you have operated for years, and it's only natural that your body will scream to go back to what has been habitual. Your mind will also play tricks on you to sidetrack your efforts—so make sure you are the boss of you. You are on a mission, and *you* are in charge. Don't give up!

Will you feel better immediately? No. I don't want to sugar coat this, so you need to know that the most common detox symptoms are headaches, light-headedness, constipation, feeling emptiness in the stomach, mild moodiness, tiredness, and even bloating. All these will go away in 2 to 5 days—I promise!

Did you know that toxicity can be addictive? When you eliminate toxins (addictive in most cases), your body will naturally respond by asking for them back. The same physiological mechanism activated when addicts go through withdrawal is what you will experience the first few days.

I can't stress enough the fact that only detrimental, unhealthy, toxic substances are addictive. Undergoing these uncomfortable side-effects is a healthy signal that repair is under way and the removal of toxins from your body is occurring. This is the time to think long–term and visualize attaining your goals. Reaching for quick, temporary relief with a candy bar, alcohol, soda, bread, or chips will get in the way of the healing detoxification process.

Watch in gratitude and amazement as your body begins this transformation. This a critical stage; don't give up now!

Prep Stage (stay here for 3 to 7 days)

This is the stage to get your body ready for going deep into the detox. You will crowd out your vices—coffee, alcohol, white carbs, processed foods, sugar, and salt—with healthier options. Take it easy on this stage and do the following:

- Reduce your coffee consumption by half. Have your reduced coffee portion after your green smoothie.
- Reduce this week's alcohol consumption by half. Or better yet, do not exceed two drinks this week.
- Replace 100% of any added sugar and artificial sweeteners with good quality stevia. A couple of drops of liquid stevia will do the trick.
- Limit all processed food to ¼ of what you are currently consuming. If you are doing the detox for 10 days, this is the time to eliminate all processed food

A typical detox day in any of the stages:

First thing in the morning: One cup of warm water with lemon

Why? Breakfast is the most important meal of the day as you are breaking a fast—a fast that your system uses to detoxify itself every night.

We want to wake up from our fast with lemon water because:

- Lemons are rich in vitamin C.
- Vitamin C enhances your beauty by rejuvenating skin from within, bringing a glow to your face.
- Lemon water paves the way for losing weight faster.
- It flushes out body toxins.
- Warm lemon water prevents constipation and diarrhea by ensuring smooth bowel functions.

In summary, lemon water is the perfect "good morning drink" as it aids the digestive system and makes the process of eliminating waste easier.

Second thing: Breakfast! A green smoothie or two or three...

Did you know that smoothies have become a controversial drink? It's because it is very easy to transform them into an unhealthy, sugary concoction. Beware of commercial smoothies full of sweeteners, all fruit, or rancid oils. The idea is to drink a super healthy drink that will keep you full for hours and meet your nutritional needs.

This quote from Dr. Joel Fuhrman, a well-respected vegan nutrition researcher and author, sums it up:

> Eating raw greens and fruits blended together to make a smooth, creamy treat is quick and convenient. The greatest benefit of blending is the increased absorption of important nutrients. All plants cells are surrounded by a cell wall that must be broken open to release the

nutrients inside. As a result, most of the valuable nutrients contained within these cells never enter our bloodstream. Blending raw, leafy greens guarantees a higher percentage of nutrients absorbed into your bloodstream. By just chewing your food you absorb about 15 – 25% of the nutrients, but blending makes your body able to absorb up to 95%!

My tips for a good detox smoothie:

- Stay away from high-glycemic fruits in your smoothies such as pineapple or mangoes. Use apple, pear, kiwi, or berries instead. If your goal includes releasing weight, I recommend using an avocado instead of a banana to ensure a creamy consistency and to reduce the sugar content.
- Keep a 4:1 ratio of vegetables to fruit.
- Optional for the prep stage: Add ground flax or chia seeds to up the fiber and protein content, slowing down sugar absorption.

You will find my favorite smoothie recipe in the recipe section. This is what I prepare for my family every morning (try all organic if possible). You can have up to 32 oz. of this nutritious drink per day.

A reminder on coffee: Reduce your intake slowly. Have your coffee after your smoothie. This way you will be crowding your tummy with nutritious liquids, thus making the urge for coffee less noticeable. Start by reducing its consumption by half and strive for elimination by the third, fifth, or seventh day depending on your detox duration.

LUNCH:

Ideally you should have a light lunch to avoid the mid-afternoon slump and to ensure a quick digestion process. Let's not make our body use more energy than needed trying to digest ill-combined foods and then expect to go back to work energized.

A few examples of easy, every day light lunches are:

- Starch Lunch 1: Big salad (any lettuce, spinach, kale, cucumbers, onions, peppers, mushrooms, olives, tomato, herbs, broccoli, or cauliflower) with one whole avocado and one baked sweet potato on the side (recipe included)
- Starch Lunch 2: Big salad and an Open-Faced Avocado Sandwich on any sprouted whole grain bread (recipe included)
- Protein-Based Lunch 1: Big salad and a Veggie Omelet (organic whole eggs, please!) (recipe included)
- Protein-Based Lunch 2: Big salad and baked salmon

Snacks:
- Left-over smoothie (keeps well in refrigerator)
- Left-over lunch (I like to make big lunches and divide them into two meals.)
- Low-sugar fresh fruit (apples, pears, any berries)
- Carrot or celery sticks with avocado or homemade Zucchini Hummus (recipe included)
- If you have a juicer, have veggie juice as a snack (I find carrot juice with ginger to be extremely comforting.)
- A handful of raw almonds
- And if very hungry, one handful of raw almonds with a banana (Make sure you wait at least 45 minutes before you eat your next meal.)

DINNERTIME:

Dinner used to be tricky for me. I was good all day but then coming home to cook for the whole family was torture. But I learned quickly that I can feed my whole family a well-combined nutritious meal that everyone will enjoy.

Take a few minutes to relax before dinner. Two to three minutes of deep belly breathing (see technique under the Consciousness Stage section) does wonders to calm you down, relax your senses, and get you ready for the nightly routine.

Always start your dinners with a salad (even just a simple plate of greens with olive oil and salt).

Main course ideas:

- Any of the lunch suggestions
- Starch Dinner: Salad and Butternut Squash Cream Soup (recipe included) If you want a heavier meal, you can also have Sautéed Veggies (recipe included) with quinoa (cook according to package).
- Protein-Based Dinner: Green salad and baked salmon with steamed broccoli

Go Stage: (stay here for 5 to 15 days)

Continue with the morning routine of lemon water and smoothie until lunch. If you are still having animal products such as red meat, pork, and chicken, this is the time to eliminate them completely. During this stage you will be dodging all coffee, alcohol, and packaged food. This will be your "Go Stage;" the temporary discomfort is gone, and you are on the go!

You will be introducing more root vegetables like sweet potatoes, carrots, beets, and other starchy veggies. Salads will be our center piece; think of the salad as the main course, not as a side dish.

Your routine will remain the same as in the prep stage, but the meal configurations will entail more organic, alkalizing greens and plant foods and less animal products. You can still eat some goat cheese, coconut and almond milk, nuts and seeds in properly combined dishes and in moderation.

Breakfast Upgrade (optional):

- If you own a juicer, upgrade your breakfast to fresh vegetable juice. My favorite recipe is Spicy Green Lemonade inspired by the talented Natalia Rose. This is my breakfast every day.

Spicy Green Lemonade (1 serving)

Ingredients:

½ bunch kale
½ head of romaine lettuce
5 celery stalks or 1 cucumber
1 whole lemon
2 inches fresh ginger
1 or 2 drops of stevia if needed for sweetness

Directions:

Pass all ingredients through the juicer following the manufacturer's instructions. Drink immediately.

Note: Juicing is a process in which an electric machine (a juicer) separates the fiber from the liquid thus creating powerful juice. Some of my clients fear that by drinking fresh veggie juice they are "wasting" the fiber. Fresh vegetable juice on an empty stomach has the ability to go straight to your cells, no digestion is needed. Because digestion is not triggered, nutrients and live enzymes drench your cells and blood immediately.

Think about a margarita versus a straight shot of tequila. Which one goes directly to your blood stream? I bet you can feel the difference, right? The same way your cells can tell the difference when you drink pure juice.

Lunch and Dinner Meal ideas:

- Make salads the principal component in every dish and follow the meal ideas listed in the Prep Stage. In this stage salads are no longer a side dish; they take center stage.

Consciousness Stage: (stay here for 2 to 6 days)

Congratulations for having made it to this point! During this stage you will be following the same guidelines as those in the Prep Stage. Continue with the morning routine of lemon water and a smoothie until lunch. By now you are familiar with food combination principles, are used to clean food, are reaping the benefits of a clean vessel, and have released some weight.

If you wish, you can re-introduce clean red meat, pork, and chicken. Make sure these are raised naturally without hormones or antibiotics or better yet, buy organic. Remember these are proteins, so combine with other foods accordingly.

I am calling this the "Consciousness Stage" because I want you to be aware, to feel, to perceive, to interpret, and most importantly to appreciate the changes that your body is experiencing. I define being conscious as being awake and aware, not on autopilot, and not doing things out of habit.

You are welcome to start playing with consciousness as early as the Prep Stage. However, I have found that one step at a time is more palpable, so I introduce this concept to my clients once they are comfortable with their new standard operating mode.

A great way to connect with yourself and become aware of your consciousness is through deep breathing. I love to do "belly breathing" (also known as diaphragmatic breathing), a wonderful calming technique. Do this every time you are about to eat or snack.

What is it? It is a simple, deep breathing technique that uses the diaphragm (below your lungs) rather than your chest to boost energy and endurance.

Follow the simple instructions below and strive for taking two or three of these breaths before every meal or snack. This will take you less than 20 seconds, and you can do it standing up, sitting down, or lying on your back.

- Start by taking a regular deep breath to relax and forget about what you are going to eat, your to do list, or other daily distractions (three to five seconds).
- Don't force this. Just focus on your breath. Start by breathing in and out through your nose at an even rate one or two times.
- Now you are ready. Put one hand on your stomach.

Take a deep breath through your nose, but now you will allow your stomach to expand, rather than your chest. You should feel the hand on your abdomen being pushed away from your body as it rises.

- Count silently to three as you inhale.
- Count silently to six as you exhale through your mouth.
- Repeat this sequence one or two more times.

Note: If you feel lightheaded, you might have been breathing too fast. Try sitting down until you get used to the surge of oxygen in your body.

Breathing and focusing your attention on the air that comes in and out, quiets your mind, releases resistance, relaxes you, and raises your consciousness.

When you are rushed and stressed, you get caught up in your head; your attention and energy feels scattered. These sensations vanish when you are focusing on the movement of your breath and the very sensations of your body. The objective is to move away from compulsive, disorganized behaviors.

■Chapter 15:
Sample Meal Plan and Yummy Recipes.

This part is geared to provide you with a few guides on menus for one week along with recipes. As long as you follow the food combination principles you can feel free to modify any of these recipes or change the order.

Many of these suggestions include items that you can cook in bulk and in advance such as quinoa, sweet potatoes, and the soups. Please keep in mind that you can make this super simple by following the food combination principles and creating your own meals using the ingredients you are comfortable with.

Remember to purchase **organic** foods. The purpose of a detox is to remove toxicants that you ingest by eating non-organic foods.

Sample Meal Plan	Monday	Tuesday	Wednesday	Thursday	Friday	Saturday
Breakfast	Green smoothie of choice	Green smoothie of choice	Green smoothie of choice	Green smoothie of choice	Green smoothie of choice	Green smoothie of choice
Lunch	Carrot/Sweet Potato Soup & Creamy Avocado Salad	Open-Faced Avocado Sandwich & green salad	Carrot/Sweet Potato Soup & Creamy Avocado Salad	Gazpacho & Open-Faced Avocado Sandwich	Veggie Omelet with green salad	Lentil Stew with green salad
Dinner	Pan Seared Scallops with Sautéed Veggies	Lemon Caper Flounder & green salad	Quinoa Salad & Butternut Squash Cream Soup	Asian Inspired Salmon with Sautéed Veggies	Open-Faced Avocado Sandwich & green salad	Asian Inspired Salmon & green salad
Snacks	Handful of unsalted raw nuts	Berry Salad	Raw Cabbage Rolls	Baked Sweet Potato	Raw veggies with Zucchini Hummus	Green apple with almond butter

Recipes:

Breakfast Smoothie

This is the base recipe. Don't be afraid to mix and match your greens and fruits. For instance, kale and chard work great in the smoothie, especially if you have a high-speed blender. Fruit options can include green apples, pears, or berries. (These fruits are easy to find in the organic or frozen sections of grocery stores.
Makes 1 serving

Ingredients:

1 cup filtered or purified water (Start with half a cup and increase as needed.)
1 head chopped, romaine lettuce
½ of large bunch of chopped, organic spinach
2 stalks of celery (only if using a high speed blender)
1 cored chopped green apple or pear, or 1c frozen berries
1 banana or avocado (I prefer avocado to avoid fruit sugars)
Juice of ½ lemon (if using high speed blender, can add 1 small, peeled lemon)
1 tablespoon of ground flax seeds and/or 1 tablespoon of chia seeds for a boost of protein and fiber (optional for prep-stage and maintenance only)

Directions:

Place all ingredients in blender. Blend until smooth.

Carrot/Sweet Potato Soup (starch)

This soup is so easy, I make a big batch and use as a snack. Makes 2 big servings and saves well for up to 5 days in a sealed glass container

Ingredients:

2 sweet potatoes
2 cups carrots
2 cups of vegetable broth
½ teaspoon sea salt
¼ teaspoon cumin
½ teaspoon coriander powder or seeds
¼ teaspoon minced ginger
1 clove of minced garlic

Directions:

Boil the sweet potatoes and carrots in the veggie broth until soft.

Put all the warm ingredients and spices in blender and process until uniform. (Please be very careful blending hot liquids.) I prefer to use an immersion blender. If you own one, then add the rest of the ingredients to the pot and blend until uniform.

Butternut Squash Cream Soup (starch)

This soup keeps well in the refrigerator. My kids have it for breakfast the next day—it's that good!
Makes 2 servings

Ingredients:

3 cloves of garlic, minced
1 yellow onion, finely chopped
1 tablespoon butter or ghee (or coconut oil if you like the taste)
2 cups of cubed butternut squash
2 cups of vegetable stock or broth
Salt and pepper to taste
1 tablespoon of olive oil

Directions:

Melt butter or ghee in large skillet over medium heat.

Sauté garlic and onion for about five minutes or until the onion becomes translucent.

Add the butternut squash, broth, salt, and pepper and let simmer until squash is tender.

With an immersion blender, blend until desired consistency. If you need more liquid, just add more broth. (If no immersion blender, then carefully transfer small amounts to a blender and blend on low speed.)

Add more salt and pepper and a drizzle of extra virgin olive oil (once all is blended) and enjoy!!!

Green Salad with Lemon Vinaigrette

Use any type of greens for this salad including spring mix, spinach, collards, kale, romaine, baby lettuces, or a combination thereof.

For the dressing:

Ingredients:

4 ounces fresh lemon juice
⅓ cup olive oil
½ teaspoon of cayenne pepper (optional)
Fine sea salt to taste
Fresh black pepper to taste

Directions:

Place all ingredients in blender. Blend until smooth.

Tahini Dressing

Ingredients:

½ cup of tahini (sesame butter)
½ cup of water
2 tablespoons of tamari
2 tablespoons of lemon juice
1 glove of garlic
1 inch of peeled, fresh ginger
3 drops of stevia

Directions:

Blend all ingredients in a blender until smooth. Add more water if needed to thin it. Note: This dressing will thicken in the fridge, and you can always add extra water to thin. You can keep this refrigerated for about 5 days.

Raw Cabbage Rolls
1 serving

Ingredients:

4 cabbage leaves (any color)
4 slices of cheddar goat cheese
Dijon mustard

Directions:

Spread a thin layer of Dijon mustard into each cabbage leaf, then add the cheese slice, roll, and enjoy. The crispiness of the cabbage pairs perfectly with the creamy combination of the cheese and mustard. Yum!

Quinoa Salad (starch)

I cook a big batch of quinoa on Sundays and set aside to be used during the week in salads or with sautéed vegetables.
Feel free to add avocado for a creamy feel and to make it a heartier meal.

Ingredients:

1 cup cooked quinoa (follow package directions)
1 cup diced tomatoes
1 cup diced, seeded cucumbers
1 cup chopped red bell peppers
1 cup chopped broccoli
1 cup diced, sweet onion
1 cup shredded carrots
1/3 of a cup of lemon vinaigrette (recipe above)

Directions:

Cook the quinoa according to the package instructions but add salt and pepper to the cooking water for taste.

In a large bowl combine quinoa and the rest of the ingredients.

Pour the lemon vinaigrette (recipe above) on top and gently toss to combine well.

Creamy Avocado Salad (starch)

Combining creamy avocado with lemon and garlic creates a luscious meal. If using this as your main meal you can use two avocados to ensure you are completely nourished and satisfied.
Makes 2 servings

Ingredients:

½ pound spring mix or baby romaine lettuce
1 medium ripe avocado, chopped
1 cup tomatoes, chopped
1 tablespoon of olive oil
2 to 3 tablespoons fresh lemon juice
1 tablespoon diced fresh garlic
3 tablespoons diced sweet onion like Vidalia
Sea salt and fresh pepper to taste

Directions:

Toss all the ingredients together in a large salad bowl, mix very well and serve.

Veggie Omelet (protein)

You can always save ¼ of this omelet and use as a snack. Saves well in the refrigerator for two days.
I like to serve this on top of a plate of fresh baby spinach.
Makes 1-2 servings

Ingredients:

4 eggs
1 cup any vegetable, chopped (This is a good time to clean your refrigerator. You can use kale, spinach, carrots, tomatoes.)
½ cup chopped onions
1 cup chopped mushrooms
1 teaspoon butter or ghee
2 slices cheddar-style goat cheese or your favorite goat cheese (optional)

Directions:

In a large bowl, whisk the eggs and set aside.

Sauté all the veggies in a pan with a little bit of water for 3 to 5 minutes. Add to eggs.

Melt the butter or ghee in the same skillet over medium heat and then add the egg mixture and cook until eggs become semi-firm.

Layer the cheese onto the eggs and fold.

Continue to cook until eggs are set.

Spanish Gazpacho (neutral)

This soup is served cold or at room temperature.   It is refreshing and will leave you wanting seconds.
Makes 2 hearty portions.

Ingredients:

1 can of fire-roasted tomatoes (or plain tomatoes if those are not available)
1 big very ripe tomato
½ diced pepper (any color)
2 cloves of garlic
The juice of one lemon
Salt and pepper to taste
2 tablespoons of extra virgin olive oil
½ diced, seeded cucumber
A bunch of parsley or basil (or both)
1 sliced avocado (optional)

Directions:

Blend all ingredients in a blender. That's it! (You can add slices of avocado on top if having a starch meal).

Open-Faced Avocado Sandwich (starch)

Simple to make yet creamy and very satisfying.
Makes 1 serving

Ingredients:

2 slices of 100% sprouted bread
1 cup diced avocado
1 tablespoon of lemon juice
2 tomato slices
A handful of baby spinach
Salt and pepper to taste

Directions:

In a mixing bowl, combine avocado, lemon, salt and pepper until all ingredients are incorporated.

Lay the spinach and tomato evenly on the two pieces of bread and spread the avocado mixture on top. Enjoy as an open-faced sandwich!

Baked Sweet Potatoes (starch)

You can cut up and add to any neutral green salad, eat cold from the fridge as a snack, or have them piping hot with butter as a main dish. Or try with butter and cinnamon for a savory snack.
4 servings

Ingredients:

4 medium-sized sweet potatoes (approximately the size of your palm).

Directions:

Preheat oven to 450°.

Scrub sweet potatoes, pat dry, and give each a few pokes with a fork, set aside.

Line cookie sheet with parchment paper and place sweet potatoes on it. Bake for approximately 1 hour.

Insert a knife after 45 minutes to ensure they are getting tender and then again at the 1 hour mark.

Once tender all the way through, they are done.

Berry Salad (fruit)

Tastes delicious if you let it stand for 30 minutes in the refrigerator. If conscious about your weight limit serving to ½ cup of berries per day.
2 servings

Ingredients:

1 cup fresh or thawed frozen blueberries
1 cup fresh or thawed frozen blackberries
1 cup fresh or thawed frozen raspberries
The juice of one lemon
3 drops of stevia

Directions:

Mix all berries in a medium bowl and set aside.

In a small bowl whisk the lemon juice and stevia.

Pour lemon mixture over berries and enjoy!

Pan Seared Scallops (protein)

2 servings

Ingredients:

1 pound large sea scallops
1 tablespoon butter
1 tablespoon coconut oil
Sea salt and freshly ground black pepper to taste
1 lemon quartered
¼ cup finely chopped herbs such as flat leaf parsley, chives, oregano, or a combination of the three.

Directions:

Wash scallops to ensure all sand is removed. Pat with paper towels until completely dry.

Heat a medium skillet (I love to use cast iron for this.) for 1 minute on high heat. Add butter and coconut oil and let them melt and get hot.

Pat scallops once more before adding to the skillet. Add them one by one and make sure they are not touching.

Season with salt and pepper and let sear 2-4 minutes per side. (Do not move the scallops except to flip them.)

Squeeze two quarters of the lemon on the scallops while they are still in the pan and sprinkle with herb mixture.

Serve ¼ of the remaining lemon with each serving.

Lemon Caper Flounder (protein)

This recipe can be made with any flaky white fish.
2 servings

Ingredients:

1 tablespoon of coconut oil
2 cloves of garlic, minced
4 flounder fillets rinsed and patted dry
2 tablespoons of capers
2 tablespoons of lemon juice
½ cup of coconut milk

Directions:

Melt the coconut oil in a large pan over high heat.

Lower heat to medium and add garlic, stir for 1 minute.

Add fish and sear carefully (1 minute each side).

Add the capers, lemon juice, and coconut milk. Stir, cover, and let simmer for 5 or 6 minutes.

Turn heat off and let the sauce thicken for two or three minutes. Serve immediately.

Sautéed Veggies (neutral)

This is a wonderful side dish or eat a big portion all by itself.
2 servings

Ingredients:

1 tablespoon sesame oil
2 cloves of garlic, minced
3 peppers, chopped (green, yellow, red)
1 cup crimini mushrooms, chopped
1 cup of broccoli or cauliflower, chopped
½ zucchini, chopped
1 teaspoon dried oregano
2 tablespoons tamari sauce
2 tablespoons of vegetable broth

Directions:

Add the sesame oil in a large sauce pan and heat on medium heat. Add garlic and sauté for one minute.

Add the remaining vegetables and cook for about two minutes.

Add the oregano, tamari sauce, and vegetable broth and stir well.

Lower the heat and let stand for three minutes.

Zucchini Humus (light protein)

I love how this lighter version feels with raw veggies.

Ingredients:

2 medium zucchinis
½ cup organic tahini
⅓ cup of lemon juice
⅓ cup of olive oil
1 teaspoon of cumin
Salt and pepper to taste

Directions:

Peel and chop the zucchinis.

Process all ingredients in a food processor (or blend at low speed in blender) until smooth.

Serve with raw veggies such as carrots, celery, broccoli, cucumber, cherry tomatoes, cauliflower, etc.

Lentil Stew (starch)

I grew up on lentil stew, yes it combines as a starch but is high in protein and fiber. One serving will leave you satiated.
2 hearty servings

Ingredients:

1 cup of dry lentils
¼ cup of olive oil
3 garlic cloves, minced
1 cup of chopped carrots
¾ cup of chopped onion
¾ cup of chopped celery
1 cup of chopped, bell peppers (any color)
3 ½ cups of veggie broth (chicken or meat broth works well also)
1-14½ oz. can of Italian stewed tomatoes
1 tablespoon of dried parsley
1 tablespoon of dried oregano
1 tablespoon of dried basil
Salt and pepper to taste

Directions:

Rinse and drain lentils.

In a saucepan, sauté the garlic, carrots, onions, celery, and bell peppers in the olive oil for five minutes.

Add the broth, tomatoes, lentils, and spices and simmer for 45 to 50 minutes until veggies and lentils are tender.

Add more salt and pepper, if desired.

Cauliflower Mash (neutral)

I never try to trick my family, but with this one I was tempted—just for the fun of it. Once you add the butter the resemblance to mashed potatoes is amazing, but cauliflower is totally neutral, full of nutrients and fiber, and easy on the stomach.
2 to 3 servings

Ingredients:

1 medium head of cauliflower. Green leaves removed.
Enough veggie or chicken broth to slightly cover cauliflower
Salt and pepper to taste
1 tablespoon butter

Directions:

Boil the cauliflower in the broth. I like to add salt to this phase for extra flavor.

Once tender, (Be careful not to overcook, we just want to soften it.) transfer to a food processor and process until the texture is exactly like mashed potatoes.
Add the butter after you achieve the desired consistency.

Check for flavor and adjust salt and pepper.

Asian Inspired Salmon

Absolutely a favorite in my house. This dish is easy and ready in no time. YUM!!
Makes 1 serving

Ingredients:

1 medium wild-caught salmon fillet
2 tablespoons tamari
1 clove of minced garlic
½ cup of finely chopped onion
1 tablespoons minced fresh ginger
1 teaspoon toasted sesame oil
1-2 drops stevia (as needed for sweetness)
1 tablespoon of toasted sesame seeds

Directions:

Mix the tamari, garlic, onion, ginger, sesame oil, and stevia in a mixing bowl to use as a marinade.

Pour the marinade over the fish (to save time do this in the same skillet you will be using).

If time allows, let this marinate in the refrigerator for a minimum of 30 minutes and up to 24 hours. (Confession: I am often pressed for time, so I put all the ingredients in a cast iron pan and cook right then and there.)

Place skillet over medium heat and cook for about 10 minutes, or until fish flakes easily with a fork.

Sprinkle toasted sesame seeds on top of the fish.

■Chapter 16:

Notes and Tips: Waste Removal, Dry Brushing, Meditation, Movement/Rest and Sexy!

A note on waste removal:

Eating plenty of plant food at every meal and eliminating the offenders listed in the "What you want to zap from your diet ASAP!" section is key to allow your body to detoxify. However, you must know that good health starts in the gut, and your efforts can be augmented when you take out all the waste. For those of you who want to take your clean state to a higher level ensuring most toxins are really leaving your body, I recommend home enemas and/or professionally administered colonics or colon hydrotherapy. A licensed colon therapist in a professional colon hydrotherapy location should only perform the later.

> Did you know that the average person has up to 10 pounds or more of dry waste in their intestine?

Let's discuss home enemas. An enema is a method used to introduce water into the colon with the intention of removing waste and stimulating bowel movements. An enema cleanses the colon by hydrating it rather than irritating it, like most common stool softeners or laxatives. Enemas have been used for many years and were a key resource used by doctors in their quest to eliminate many ailments.

Ok, now that you know the benefits of an enema, please don't discard their use, run away, or close this book. I know that the thought of inserting a catheter up your rectum might not sound appealing at all, but an enema can and should be part of your cleansing routine and can be a nurturing experience.

Whenever you feel constipated, heavy in your intestines, or full of gas, it is time for an enema. However, as you continue your quest for a healthier lifestyle, enemas should be part of your routine even when you feel great.

I personally use the kit with the stainless bucket instead of the typical enema bag for ease of use and super easy cleanup. I only recommend doing the enema with filtered water; nothing else is needed to perfectly hydrate the colon. There are many how-to videos available on the internet. Carefully follow the instructions and enjoy the benefits!

A note on dry skin brushing:

The skin is the largest organ in the body and carries one fourth of the task of daily detoxification. So with that impressive job description, we cannot ignore it.

Did you know that the skin eliminates an average of two pounds of waste every day?

Dry skin brushing is one of the best methods to assist in the detoxification and toning of the skin. Dry brushing helps shed dead skin cells, increases circulation, aids the lymphatic drainage, tightens the skin by increasing blood flow, lessens the appearance of cellulite, stimulates the nerve endings of the skin, and it feels great especially before showering or in the morning.

I recommend only 100% natural vegetable bristle brushes, which are sold in healthy supermarkets, health stores, and on line for less than $12.00.

Skin brushing is super simple and should be performed once a day in the morning on a naked body. Begin brushing in long sweeps beginning from your feet upwards (as if you were shaving your legs) and then do the same starting from your hands. Always brush towards your heart and avoid any sensitive areas. It takes me no more than one minute to brush my legs, arms, and tummy two or three times every morning.

A note on meditation:

Meditation is beneficial but also easy—you do not need any equipment, you can do it anywhere, it takes about five minutes (for beginners), and it is free. It can't get much simpler than that!

I consider myself blessed for having found the powerful tool of meditation. I used to think meditation was not for me; I was too busy and too stressed to bother, and my mind was always full of thoughts and ideas. How could I stop all that? Well, it just so happens that somebody like me is the perfect person to meditate for various reasons.

All you need to do is find a quiet place and get in a comfortable seated position. Now focus all your attention on the flow of your breath. In and out, follow your breath, easy effortlessly. Every day when I start meditating I ask, What do I want? What do I really want today? Sometimes I have the answer and sometimes I don't, but I ask anyway and let the universe take care of it. And you know what? The universe always does (ask and you shall receive). It's that simple—ask and follow your breath. If your thoughts invade your head, let them. Don't fight them, simply keep following your breaths. As you get comfortable you will want to increase your time.

A recent comprehensive scientific study was performed at Harvard Medical School. This research found that meditation practiced regularly helps enhance the genes that help fight disease and reduce stress. Stress releases stress-hormones such as cortisol and adrenaline, which raise blood pressure, compromise immunity, make us retain fat, and feel exhausted for no reason. So if meditation lowers stress, it is only normal that it will produce feel-good chemicals such as serotonin, lower blood pressure, boost immunity, and allow us to thrive in our body.

Five minutes per day, that is all it takes.

A Note on Movement and Rest:

Movement and rest might initially seem to be opposites, but when you are in the process of detoxifying your body, they are on the same spectrum.

During detox you want to encourage toxins to "move" out. You do this by pairing movement with eating more greens and unprocessed food and drinking more water. This combination improves the efficiency of the program.

Simple, easy, and fun movement is what I want you to

incorporate into your routine. Make sure you do not overdo it. My favorite ways to move while on a detox include yoga, Pilates, stretching, hiking, easy biking, and even walking around the neighborhood. Feel free to try whatever feels right for you. If you like swimming or tai chi, for example, go for it. Daily movement will aide your lymphatic system in the detoxification process.

On the other side of the spectrum is rest—a full eight hours per day minimum rest and sleep. Rest is the tool that will allow your body to restore itself and enable you to move more the next day.

Adequate daily rest is key to detoxification, but you still work way too many hours and feel guilty when you take it easy. The body, the mind, and the spirit repair and strengthen when you rest. Adequate rest will result in better mental alertness the next day, thus making you more efficient. Generally speaking, adequate rest and sleep will help maintain better balance between personal, professional, and family life.

Not getting enough rest results in mysterious changes in hormone levels such as cortisol (your stress regulator), lower levels of activity of human growth hormone (which repairs tissue), declined aerobic resistance, and an amplified unrealistic sense of exertion.

In summary, being aware of the relationship between movement and rest to your hormonal balance and making changes in your routine to improve in these areas is key to managing the changes associated with the "pause of meno."

A Tip on *Sexy!* as Defined by 100 Men:

Many of my clients who are around fifty years old want to be sexy, love the topic, but deep down believe that sexy is not for them. Even though I find them all beautiful, it seems that what they define as sexy is unattainable. They are convinced that sexy is for younger women, svelte-type models that only appear on TV and magazines.

So I decided to start my own research to re-define sexy. I interviewed one hundred fabulous men of all ages, from thirteen years old to eighty-four, and one hundred percent of these individuals agreed on one thing—confidence is sexy. One hundred percent said this!!!

When I asked them, what is "sexy" to you? Their responses were almost identical and included phrases such as: "confident," "sexy is ageless," "a woman who knows what she wants," "independent," "knows how to dress for her size," "acts her age," "asks for what she wants," "comfortable and honest," "warm and real." Sexy is "found in the little things...pulling her hair back to show her neck, ears, jewelry," "wearing a nice flowing dress," "a sense of humor," "being accepting of her body regardless her size," and "a woman that loves herself is sexy."

The most beautiful definition came from my friend Dr. Jonathan Wasserman:

> A sexy woman truly runs the gamut across many spectrums. Sure, the alluring clothing, shoes, make-up, hair and exposed undergarments can add to an external shell of, "Hey look me over!" But in my world, sexy isn't the perfect body or

glamorous make-up or deeply exposed cleavage.

Intelligence can be sexy, as can confidence, success, and independence. But it is the woman who is confident with who she is, comfortable with how she is, and loves and accepts herself who is the sexiest. Sexy should first exude from within, from the eyes, the smile, and the ability to maintain a balanced conversation. A truly sexy woman will also appreciate those same factors in her partner(s), as well as acknowledge that person. For if she can find and observe it in others, that in itself, is the moment of enlightenment that she owns those characteristics herself.

Closing thoughts:

Amazing shifts started happening in my life when I decided to take control of those things I do have power over instead of craving control over those I don't. At my age and facing the preparatory stages for the "pause of meno" (or menopause) too much of a good thing can throw me off balance, and that is not how I want to live the second half of my life.

It took me several years of research and experiments in my own body to feel great today. I am never tired, and I rest peacefully at night. My sugar and carb cravings disappeared. I have an occasional glass of red wine with my friends and family but never to relax, to forget, loosen up, or be able to fall asleep.

Ladies, this is our time to enjoy maturity at our best. Wouldn't you love to be at home in your body, crave good food, love moving your body, be aroused often, and feel sexier than ever? This is what I want for you, and this book is the first step to get you there. Allow yourself this gift today.

REFERENCES

Academy of Environmental Medicine; "Genetically Modified Foods," study by Amy Dean, O.D. and Jennifer Armstrong, M.D., May 8, 2009, http://www.aaemonline.org/gmopost.html.

Center for Disease Control, *Fourth National Report on Human Exposure to Environmental Chemicals,* last modified September 2012, http://www.cdc.gov/exposurereport/pdf/FourthReport.pdf.

Colquhoun, James, and Laurentine Ten Bosch. *Hungry for Change: Ditch the Diets, Conquer the Cravings, and Eat Your Way to Lifelong Health.* New York: Harper One (2012): 86-7.

Dietary Supplement Health and Education Act of 1994, Pub. L. No. 103-417, 108 Stat. 4325 (1994).

"Eat to Live What's Cooking?," Dr. Joel Fuhrman, last modified March 2006, http://www.drfuhrman.com/library/bulletin/March_Recipe_Newsletter.html

Environmental Working Group, The Online, s.v. "Dirty Dozen™ Plus," last modified April 2014, http://www.ewg.org/foodnews/summary.php.

Federal Drug Administration, *Food and Drug Administration on Compliance Program Guidance Manual 7304.019,* last modified October 30, 2010, http://www.fda.gov/downloads/food/guidancecomplianceregulatoryinformation/complianceenforcement/ucm073204.pdf

Harvard Health Publications Harvard Medical School; "Mindful Meditation May Ease Anxiety, Mental Stress," article by Julie Corliss, January 8, 2014, http://www.health.harvard.edu/blog/mindfulness-meditation-may-ease-anxiety-mental-stress-201401086967.

Lee, John R., and Virginia Hopkins. *What Your Doctor May Not Tell You About Menopause.* New York: Warner Books, 2004.

National Institute for Environmental Health Sciences Online, s.v. "endocrine disruptors," last modified July 18, 2014, http://www.niehs.nih.gov/health/topics/agents/endocrine/.

National Toxicology Program Online, s.v. "aloe vera testing," last modified August 2013, http://ntp.niehs.nih.gov/results/pubs/longterm/reports/longter m/tr500580/listedreports/tr577/index.html

Rose, Natalia. *Detox for Women*. New York: William Morrow, 2009.

———. *The Raw Food Detox Diet*. New York: Regan, 2005.
Snyder, Kimberly. *The Beauty Detox Solution*. Ontario: Harlequin, 2011.

Merriam-Webster Online, s.v. "pollution," accessed August 8, 2010, http://merriam-webster.com/dictionary/pollution.

Million Women Study Online, s.v. "hormone replacement study," last modified December 2012, http://www.millionwomenstudy.org/study_progress/.

U.S. Department of Health and Human Services Online, s.v. "constipation," last modified May 28, 2014, http://digestive.niddk.nih.gov/ddiseases/pubs/constipation/.

U.S. Food and Drug Administration Online, s.v. "Biotechnology Genetically Engineered Food and Feed," last modified May 31, 2013, http://www.fda.gov/Food/FoodScienceResearch/Biotechnology/d efault.htm.

———, s.v. "Generally Recognized as Safe (GRAS) Notification Program," last modified June 19, 2014, http://www.fda.gov/animalveterinary/products/animalfoodfeeds /generallyrecognizedassafegrasnotifications/default.htm.

———, s.v. "What is the meaning of 'natural' on the label of food?," last modified April 10, 2014, http://www.fda.gov/aboutfda/transparency/basics/ucm214868.htm.

Women's Health Initiative, *Findings from the WHI Postmenopausal Hormone Replacement Trials,* last modified January 12, 2010, http://www.nhlbi.nih.gov/whi/.

ABOUT THE AUTHOR

Mari Carmen Pizarro is a best selling author, certified holistic health, health and nutrition, and master transformational coach, as well as a board-certified, fully accredited member of the American Association of Drugless Practitioners.

Mari Carmen completed her MBA requirements and maintained a successful career as a senior human resources leader for more than twenty years. But even as her career was flourishing, her physical health was diminishing, and she wanted to find a way to control it.

In 2006, Mari Carmen made dramatic changes in both her career and lifestyle, and indeed, she did find a way to control her health. Through her subsequent work, she has helped countless other women achieve the same results.

Now you, too, can benefit from Mari Carmen's passion, expertise, and knowledge, as shared in this inspiring book, Gone in a Flash!

For more information about other programs or to work with Mari Carmen directly please visit her website at www.StreamlinedHealth.com .

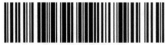

Made in the USA
San Bernardino, CA
16 March 2016